PCOS WEIGHT LOSS COOKBOOK

Fight and win polycystic ovarian syndrome by weight reduction, with delicious and time saving recipes and meal plan.

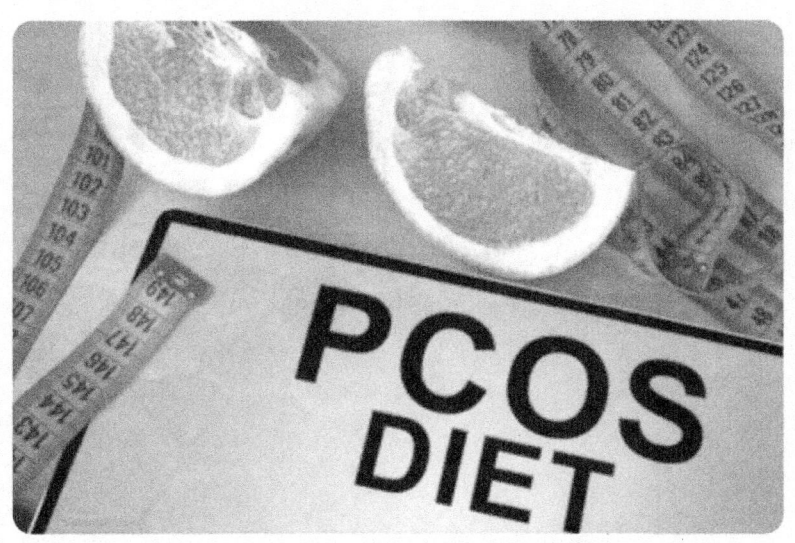

Jenny Rick

Copyright © 2023 by Jenny Rick

All rights reserved. No part of this publication may be reproduced, distributed, or transmitted in any form or by any means, including photocopying, recording, or other electronic or mechanical methods, without the prior written permission of the publisher, except in the case of brief quotations embodied in critical reviews and certain other non commercial uses permitted by copyright law.

Table of Contents

INTRODUCTION	19
CHAPTER ONE	23
Polycystic Ovarian Syndrome	23
CHAPTER TWO	25
Understanding PCOS and weight loss	25
CHAPTER THREE	27
Nutrition Basics for PCOS Weight Loss	27
CHAPTER FOUR	29
PCOS-Friendly Meal Planning	29
BREAKFAST	31
1. Overnight Oats with Fresh Fruit	31
2. Egg Muffins	31
3. Sweet Potato Toast	31
4. Broccoli and Cheese Egg Muffins	31
5. Peanut Butter Banana Protein Smoothie	32
6. Greek Yogurt Parfait	32
7. Avocado Toast	32
8. Egg and Avocado Wrap	32
9. Apple Pie Overnight Oats	32
10. Egg and Vegetable Bake	33
11. Savory Oatmeal	33
12. Sweet Potato Hash	33

13. Egg and Vegetable Frittata 33
14. Apple Walnut Oatmeal 34
15. Greek Yogurt Bowl 34
16. Banana Protein Pancakes 34
17. Vegetable and Egg White Omelet 34
18. Egg and Spinach Sandwich 35
19. Almond Butter Banana Toast 35
20. Protein Power Bowl 35
21. Green Smoothie Bowl 35
22. PB&J Overnight Oats 36
23. Chia Pudding 36
24. Egg, Spinach, and Tomato Breakfast Wrap 36
25. Protein Pancakes with Berries 36
26. Egg and Veggie Breakfast Burrito 37
27. Overnight Oats with Apple 37
28. Greek Yogurt and Fruit Bowl 37
29. Avocado Egg Toast 37
30. Chia Seed Pudding with Berries 38
31. Zucchini Muffins 38
32. Spinach and Feta Egg Muffins 38
33. Oatmeal with Nuts and Fruit 38
34. Broccoli and Cheese Frittata 39
35. Sweet Potato and Egg Hash 39

36. Protein Waffles 39

37. Greek Yogurt with Nuts and Fruit 40

38. Apple Cinnamon Protein Pancakes 40

39. Zucchini Fritters 40

40. Protein Oatmeal 40

41. Baked Egg Cups 41

42. Egg and Veggie Breakfast Bowl 41

43. Almond Butter Overnight Oats 41

44. Avocado Toast with Egg 41

45. Baked Apple 42

46. Kale and Feta Egg Muffins 42

47. Quinoa Breakfast Bowl 42

48. Smoothie Bowl 42

49. Egg and Avocado Breakfast Sandwich 43

50. Protein French Toast 43

51. Baked Sweet Potato 43

52. Omelet with Veggies 43

53. Egg and Veggie Breakfast Pizza 44

54. Banana Oat Greek Yogurt 44

55. Carrot Cake Overnight Oats 44

56. Protein Toast 44

57. Sweet Potato Hash with Eggs 44

58. Green Smoothie 45

59. Baked Oatmeal 45
60. Protein Pancakes with Nuts and Fruit 45
61. Egg Muffins with Veggies 46
62. Blueberry Protein Pancakes 46
63. Oatmeal Breakfast Bars 46
64. Vegetable Omelet 46
65. Baked Egg Cups with Vegetables 47
66. Peanut Butter Banana Smoothie 47
67. Sweet Potato Toast with Avocado 47
68. Zucchini Fritters with Avocado 47
69. Apple Pie Oatmeal 48
70. Egg, Spinach, and Tomato Breakfast Bowl 48
71. Baked Apples with Nuts and Seeds 48
72. Sweet Potato Toast with Egg 49
73. Blue Smoothie Bowl 49
74. Banana Walnut Protein Pancakes 49
75. Egg and Veggie Breakfast Wrap 49
76. Quinoa Porridge 50
77. Avocado Toast with Tomatoes 50
78. Kale and Feta Egg Cups 50
79. Apple Cinnamon Oatmeal 51
80. Mashed Sweet Potato Toast 51
81. Strawberry Protein Pancakes 51

82. Broccoli and Cheese Frittata 51

83. Banana Nut Butter Smoothie 52

84. Oatmeal with Nuts and Seeds 52

85. Blueberry Overnight Oats 52

86. Avocado Toast with Egg and Spinach 52

87. Zucchini Bread 52

88. Egg and Veggie Breakfast Burrito Bowl 53

89. Protein French toast with Berries 53

91. Egg and Avocado Breakfast Sandwich 54

93. Quinoa Breakfast Burrito 54

94. Baked Sweet Potato with Nuts and Seeds 54

95. Protein Oatmeal with Berries 55

96. Avocado Egg Toast with Spinach 55

97. Egg and Veggie Breakfast Sandwich 55

98. Blueberry Coconut Oatmeal 56

99. Kale and Feta Egg Wrap 56

100. Protein Waffles with Nuts and Fruit 56

LUNCH 57

101. Roasted Vegetable Wrap 57

102. Quinoa Bowl 57

103. Mediterranean Salad 57

104. Deli Roll-Ups 57

105. Wild Salmon Salad 58

106. Turkey Sandwich 58
107. Peanut Butter and Banana Sandwich 58
108. Baked Egg Wrap 58
109. Veggie Burger 58
110. Zucchini Noodles 59
111. Avocado Toast 59
112. Tuna Salad 59
113. Spinach Salad 59
114. Mexican Rice Bowl 59
115. Cucumber Sandwich 59
116. Lentil Soup 60
117. Turkey and Veggie Skewers 60
118. Quinoa Stuffed Peppers 60
119. Curried Chicken Salad 60
120. Cobb Salad 60
121. Kale and Quinoa Bowl 60
122. Asian Noodle Bowl 61
123. Egg Salad 61
124. Hummus and Veggie Wrap 61
125. Greek Salad 61
126. Tuna Melt 61
127. Avocado Egg Salad 62
128. Mediterranean Chicken Wrap 62

129. Broccoli and Cheese Omelet 62
130. Turkey and Veggie Sandwich 62
131. Lentil and Vegetable Soup 62
132. Baked Sweet Potato 62
133. Quinoa and Veggie Salad 63
134. Egg and Avocado Toast 63
135. Turkey and Quinoa Bowl 63
136. Fruit Salad 63
137. Vegetable Soup 63
138. Bacon, Spinach, and Cheese Wrap 63
139. Falafel Wrap 64
140. Greek Yogurt Parfait 64
141. Chicken Salad Sandwich 64
142. Quinoa and Black Bean Burrito 64
143. Tuna and Avocado Salad 64
144. Grilled Vegetables 64
145. Roasted Eggplant Sandwich 65
146. Egg and Vegetable Frittata 65
147. Chickpea Salad 65
148. Chicken and Rice Bowl 65
149. Avocado and Egg Toast 65
150. Mango Smoothie 65
151. Tomato and Mozzarella Sandwich 66

152. Hummus and Veggie Sandwich 66

153. Curry Bowl 66

154. Tofu and Veggie Stir-Fry 66

155. Salmon and Rice Bowl 66

156. Zucchini Fritters 66

157. Egg and Cheese Sandwich 67

158. Fruit Salad Bowl 67

159. Turkey and Cheese Sandwich 67

160. Lentil Salad 67

161. Baked Potato 67

162. Egg and Avocado Wrap 67

163. Veggie Omelet 68

164. Quinoa-Stuffed Peppers 68

165. Greek Salad Bowl 68

166. BBQ Chicken Sandwich 68

167. Chickpea and Vegetable Wrap 68

168. Tomato Soup 68

169. Roasted Vegetable Sandwich 69

170. Fruit and Yogurt Bowl 69

171. Egg Salad Wrap 69

172. Turkey and Cheese Wrap 69

173. Lentil and Rice Bowl 69

174. Quinoa and Black Bean Salad 69

175. Vegetable and Cheese Omelet 70
176. Baked Sweet Potato and Bean Burrito 70
177. Turkey Burger 70
178. Mediterranean Quinoa Bowl 70
179. Grilled Cheese Sandwich 70
180. Greek Yogurt Parfait 71
181. Baked Potato and Egg 71
182. Tofu Scramble 71
183. Hummus and Veggie Toast 71
184. Egg and Vegetable Frittata 71
185. Chicken and Rice Soup 71
186. Curry Bowl 72
187. Tuna and Avocado Wrap 72
188. Quinoa and Vegetable Salad 72
189. Turkey and Veggie Sandwich 72
190. Egg and Cheese Wrap 72
191. Baked Eggplant Sandwich 72
192. Lentil Soup 73
193. Mango Smoothie 73
194. Falafel Wrap 73
195. Chickpea Salad 73
196. Baked Potato and Bean Burrito 73
197. Vegetable Soup 73

198. Tofu and Veggie Stir-Fry 73

199. Avocado Toast 74

200. Curried Chicken Salad 74

DINNER 75

201. Mediterranean Quinoa Bowl 75

202. Veggie Stir Fry 75

203. Grilled Chicken Salad 75

204. Turkey and Veggie Burgers 75

205. Roasted Veggie and Quinoa Bowl 76

206. Grilled Salmon with Asparagus 76

207. Baked Tilapia with Sweet Potato 76

208. Eggplant Parmesan 76

209. Turkey Chili 77

210. Zucchini Noodles with Avocado Pesto 77

211. Baked Tilapia with Roasted Tomatoes 77

212. Turkey Taco Salad 77

213. Baked Salmon with Broccoli 78

214. Quinoa Salad 78

215. Baked Eggplant Parmesan 78

216. Grilled Vegetable Skewers 78

217. Turkey and Veggie Stuffed Peppers 79

218. Roasted Potato and Chickpea Salad 79

219. Baked Fish with Spinach 79

220. Sweet Potato Fries 79

221. Grilled Halibut with Mango Salsa 80

222. Quinoa Veggie Burgers 80

223. Baked Cod with Roasted Broccoli 80

224. Baked Tofu with Asparagus 80

225. Lentil Soup 80

226. Grilled Chicken with Roasted Vegetables 81

227. Baked Eggplant and Quinoa Casserole 81

228. Turkey and Kale Stuffed Sweet Potatoes 81

229. Grilled Zucchini Boats 82

230. Baked Salmon with Spaghetti Squash 82

231. Zucchini Lasagna 82

232. Eggplant and Quinoa Stuffed Peppers 82

233. Grilled Portobello Mushrooms 83

234. Baked Tilapia with Roasted Asparagus 83

235. Salad Niçoise 83

236. Veggie Fajitas 83

237. Baked Sweet Potato Fries 84

238. Grilled Salmon with Spinach 84

239. Baked Tofu with Quinoa 84

240. Roasted Vegetable Soup 84

241. Lentil Tacos 84

242. Turkey and Quinoa Sliders 85

243. Baked Eggplant Parmesan 85
244. Vegetable Curry 85
245. Grilled Halibut with Mango Salsa................................85
246. Stuffed Zucchini 86
247. Cauliflower Rice Bowl 86
248. Baked Tilapia with Broccoli 86
249. Baked Eggplant with Quinoa.......................................86
250. Grilled Shrimp with Roasted Vegetables 87
251. Baked Sweet Potato Fries 87
252. Eggplant and Lentil Curry..87
253. Quinoa Bowl with Roasted Vegetables......................87
254. Baked Fish with Asparagus 88
255. Grilled Vegetable and Quinoa Salad 88
256. Baked Eggplant Parmesan 88
257. Lentil and Veggie Burgers 88
258. Grilled Salmon with Sautéed Spinach 89
259. Baked Tofu with Broccoli 89
260. Zucchini Noodles with Avocado Pesto 89
261. Mediterranean Quinoa Bowl 89
262. Eggplant and Quinoa Casserole 89
263. Baked Cod with Roasted Asparagus...........................90
264. Grilled Vegetable Skewers 90
265. Baked Tilapia with Roasted Tomatoes.......................90

266. Baked Salmon with Roasted Potatoes 91
267. Quinoa and Veggie Stir Fry 91
268. Turkey Chili 91
269. Grilled Chicken Salad 91
270. Baked Eggplant with Lentils 92
271. Lentil Soup 92
272. Grilled Portobello Mushrooms 92
273. Vegetable Curry 92
274. Baked Tilapia with Broccoli 93
275. Quinoa Bowl with Roasted Vegetables 93
276. Baked Salmon with Spinach 93
277. Baked Tofu with Roasted Vegetables 93
278. Baked Eggplant with Quinoa 94
279. Grilled Shrimp with Roasted Tomatoes 94
280. Lentil and Veggie Burgers 94
281. Baked Tofu with Broccoli 94
282. Mediterranean Quinoa Bowl 95
283. Eggplant and Quinoa Casserole 95
284. Grilled Salmon with Sautéed Spinach 95
285. Baked Cod with Roasted Asparagus 95
286. Baked Eggplant Parmesan 96
287. Grilled Vegetable Skewers 96
288. Baked Tilapia with Roasted Tomatoes 96

289. Baked Salmon with Roasted Potatoes 96

290. Quinoa and Veggie Stir Fry...97

291. Turkey Chili 97

292. Grilled Chicken Salad: Grill 2 chicken breasts 97

293. Baked Eggplant with Lentils 97

294. Lentil Soup 98

295. Grilled Portobello Mushrooms 98

296. Vegetable Curry 98

297. Zucchini Noodles with Avocado Pesto 98

298. Cauliflower Rice Bowl 99

299. Baked Sweet Potato Fries 99

300. Eggplant and Lentil Curry..99

DESERT 100

301. Quinoa Salad with Feta and Pomegranate 100

302. Avocado and Mango Salad..100

303. Grilled Eggplant and Zucchini Skewers 100

304. Stuffed Peppers with Quinoa..100

305. Grilled Vegetable Platter...101

306. Chickpea and Spinach Curry..101

307. Sweet Potato Fries 101

308. Mediterranean Baked Fish..101

309. Eggplant Parmesan 102

310. Quinoa Pilaf..102

SNACKS 104

311. Baked Apples with Cinnamon 104

312. Avocado Toast with Poached Egg 104

313. Kale Chips 104

314. Baked Sweet Potato Fries 104

315. Cucumber Slices with Hummus 104

316. Baked Zucchini Coins with Parmesan 105

317. Roasted Chickpeas 105

318. Greek Yogurt with Berries 105

319. Apple Slices with Almond Butter 105

320. Celery with Peanut Butter 105

321. Roasted Eggplant Rounds 105

322. Popcorn with Coconut Oil 106

323. Baked Tofu Fries 106

324. Baked Potato Wedges 106

325. Baked Kale Chips 106

326. Avocado Egg Salad 106

327. Baked Plantain Chips 106

328. Roasted Cauliflower 107

329. Greek Yogurt with Granola 107

330. Zucchini Noodles with Pesto 107

CHAPTER FIVE 109

Meal Preparation Tips and Strategies 109

CHAPTER SIX 111
    PCOS friendly exercises for weight loss 111
CONCLUSION 113

INTRODUCTION

Are you looking for a way to lose weight and manage the symptoms of PCOS? You're not alone.

Polycystic Ovary Syndrome (PCOS) is one of the most common endocrine disorders in women of reproductive age, and it can cause a wide range of symptoms including weight gain, infertility, and hair loss.

If you're struggling with PCOS, you may have tried a variety of diets and treatments to help manage your symptoms. But have you considered the potential benefits of cooking for PCOS? Cooking for PCOS can be a great way to lose weight, manage your symptoms, and improve your overall health. That's why I have written the PCOS Cookbook for Weight Loss.

Inside, you'll find delicious, nutritious recipes designed to help you achieve your goals. I've also provide you with tips and strategies to make cooking for PCOS easier and more enjoyable. So, whether you're just starting out or you're an experienced cook, this cookbook will help you find the right meal plan for you.

It contains delicious and time saving recipes to help make your PCOS journey a success. With this cookbook, you will learn how to make healthier choices and create a diet that can help you lose weight, while still keeping your PCOS in check.

I want to share with you some inspiring stories from people who have found success in managing their PCOS through dieting and weight loss. Read on to learn more about their journey and find out how you can follow in their footsteps.

Sarah: Eighteen year old Sarah was diagnosed of pcos by her family gynecologist few years back. Being overweight she was advised by her doctor to lose some weight as this will help with managing her pcos symptoms. Sarah found this idea so challenging since it might entail having to quiet some of her best meals and snacks. Enshrouded with the thoughts that dieting ultimately means eating little portions of some tasteless vegetables and every other thing an eighteen years old wouldn't want to, she started being depressed about her condition. Few months into talking with her and sharing recipes from this book with her, Sarah was able to lose 15 pounds. Judging from where she was coming from that is some serious progress to be proud of. Sarah commended that the recipes weren't tasteless and she got to enjoy new good meals while shedding some weight. She was amazed at the results and has been able to keep the weight off for over a year!

Jennifer: Jennifer a colleague of mine was diagnosed with PCOS just a few months ago and was scared of the potential weight gain. Sharing recipes from this book with her, she was able to make changes to her diet and this helped her keep the weight off and even lose a few pounds. She's been able to maintain her weight and keep her PCOS symptoms under control.

If Sarah and Jennifer can do it then you too can!
Come along with me as I share with you proven delicious recipes that will help you lose some weight and keep your PCOS symptoms under control.

With the right tools and this cookbook, you can achieve the same level of success. So let's get cooking!

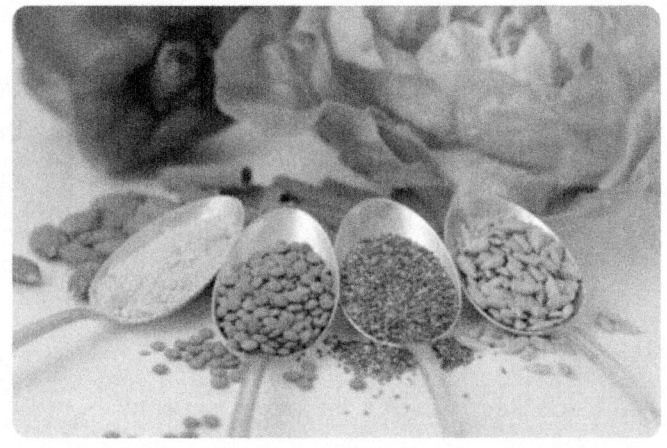

CHAPTER ONE

Polycystic Ovarian Syndrome

Polycystic Ovary Syndrome (PCOS) is a common hormonal disorder that affects women of reproductive age, and is one of the leading causes of female infertility. It is a complex disorder that affects women in a variety of ways, including physical, emotional, and psychological.

PCOS is caused by an imbalance of hormones, including an elevated level of androgens (male hormones), which can lead to the formation of multiple small cysts on the ovaries.

The exact cause of PCOS is unknown, but several factors may be involved, including genetics, insulin resistance, inflammation, and environmental factors. Symptoms of PCOS can vary from woman to woman, but the most common symptoms include irregular or absent menstrual periods, excessive facial and body hair growth, acne, and weight gain.

PCOS is a lifelong condition, but there are treatments available to help manage the symptoms. Treatment options typically involve lifestyle changes, such as dietary changes, increased physical activity, and weight loss, as well as medical treatments such as hormone therapy, medications, and surgery.

Women with PCOS can also benefit from support and counseling to help manage the condition. It is important for women with PCOS to be aware of their risk of developing other conditions, such as diabetes, high blood pressure, and cardiovascular disease.

Although there is no cure for PCOS, it is possible to manage the condition and live a healthy and productive life. It is important for women to talk to a healthcare provider about their symptoms and treatment options. With proper diagnosis and treatment, women with PCOS can live a normal, healthy life.

CHAPTER TWO

Understanding PCOS and weight loss

Polycystic ovarian syndrome (PCOS) is a common endocrine disorder in women of reproductive age that can cause a wide range of symptoms, including irregular menstrual cycles, excessive hair growth, acne, and infertility. It can also lead to weight gain, which can be a difficult side effect to manage.

Weight loss is possible with PCOS, but it may require a combination of lifestyle changes, such as increasing physical activity, eating a healthy balanced diet, and managing stress.

Reducing refined carbohydrates and sugars, eating more high-fiber foods, and focusing on nutrient-dense options, such as lean proteins and healthy fats, can also help. It is important to remember that weight loss, while beneficial in reducing PCOS symptoms, can be difficult to achieve and maintain.

It is best to work with a healthcare provider to come up with a safe and effective plan of action that takes into account your individual needs and goals.

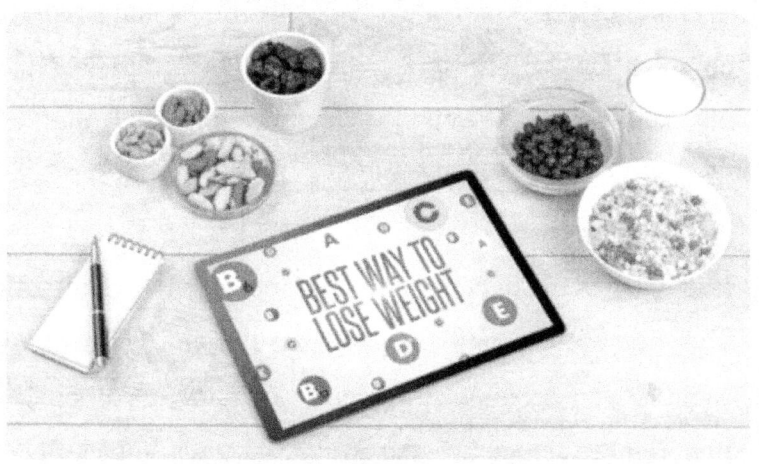

CHAPTER THREE

Nutrition Basics for PCOS Weight Loss

1. Eat a balanced diet: Consume a balanced diet that includes a variety of nutrient-dense foods such as lean proteins, healthy fats, fruits, vegetables, whole grains and dairy.

2. Eat enough calories: Eating too few calories can lead to weight gain and make it harder to lose weight. Aim to eat enough calories to meet your energy needs, but not so much that you gain weight.

3. Limit processed and refined foods: Processed and refined foods are often high in added sugars and unhealthy fats, which can lead to weight gain. Choose whole foods as much as possible.

4. Choose high-fiber foods: High-fiber foods, such as fruits, vegetables, whole grains and legumes, can help you feel full and reduce your risk of overeating.

5. Get enough protein: Protein helps build muscle and can help you feel full, making it easier to stick to a healthy diet. Aim for at least 0.8g of protein per kilogram of body weight each day.

6. Avoid sugary drinks and snacks: Sugary drinks and snacks can add a lot of empty calories to your diet, making it harder to lose weight. Choose water and unsweetened drinks instead.

7. Be mindful of portion sizes: Eating large portions can lead to overeating and weight gain. Use smaller plates and bowls to help control your portions.

8. Move more: Exercise is essential for PCOS weight loss. Aim for at least 150 minutes of moderate-intensity exercise each week.

CHAPTER FOUR
PCOS-Friendly Meal Planning

PCOS-friendly meal planning involves making dietary changes to help manage the symptoms of polycystic ovary syndrome (PCOS).

The goal of PCOS-friendly meal planning is to lower androgen levels, balance hormones, reduce inflammation, and support fertility.

A PCOS-friendly meal plan should include plenty of fresh fruits and vegetables, lean proteins, and healthy fats, as well as complex carbohydrates such as whole grains, legumes, and starchy vegetables.

Eating several small meals throughout the day can help keep blood sugar levels stable, which can help reduce symptoms of PCOS.

It is also important to reduce or eliminate processed and refined foods, sugary beverages, and trans fats from the diet.

Eating a variety of foods and limiting processed foods can help reduce inflammation and support a healthy weight. In addition to dietary changes, being physically active can help improve symptoms of PCOS and reduce the risk of developing metabolic disorders.

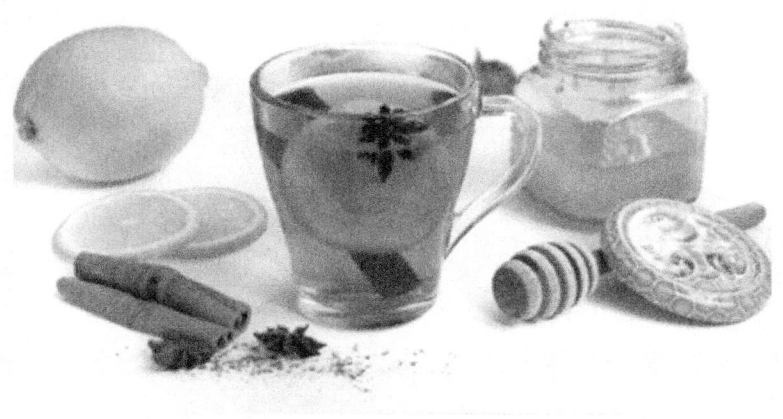

BREAKFAST

1. Overnight Oats with Fresh Fruit:

Combine rolled oats, chia seeds, and almond milk in a mason jar. Let sit overnight in the refrigerator, then top with your favorite fresh fruit in the morning.

2. Egg Muffins:

Preheat oven to 350°F. Grease a muffin tin with coconut oil. Whisk together eggs, diced onions, bell peppers, and your favorite herbs and spices. Divide egg mixture into muffin tin and bake for 20-25 minutes, or until eggs are cooked through. Enjoy with a side of fresh fruit.

3. Sweet Potato Toast:

Spread mashed sweet potato on toasted whole grain bread. Top with a sprinkle of cinnamon and a drizzle of honey.

4. Broccoli and Cheese Egg Muffins:

Preheat oven to 375°F. Grease a muffin tin with coconut oil. Whisk together eggs, shredded broccoli, and shredded cheese. Divide egg mixture into muffin tin and bake for 20-25 minutes, or until eggs are cooked through. Enjoy with a side of fresh fruit.

5. Peanut Butter Banana Protein Smoothie:

Blend together 1 banana, 1 scoop of protein powder, 1 tablespoon of peanut butter, and ¾ cup of almond milk. Enjoy with a sprinkle of chia seeds and cinnamon.

6. Greek Yogurt Parfait:

Layer low-fat Greek yogurt, fresh fruit, and your favorite granola in a bowl. Top with a drizzle of honey.

7. Avocado Toast:

Spread mashed avocado on toasted whole grain bread. Top with a sprinkle of sea salt and a drizzle of olive oil.

8. Egg and Avocado Wrap:

Spread mashed avocado on a whole grain tortilla. Top with scrambled egg and your favorite herbs and spices. Roll up and enjoy.

9. Apple Pie Overnight Oats:

Combine rolled oats, chia seeds, almond milk, diced apples, and a sprinkle of cinnamon in a mason jar. Let sit overnight in the refrigerator, then top with your favorite nuts in the morning.

10. Egg and Vegetable Bake:

Preheat oven to 400°F. Grease a baking dish with coconut oil. Whisk together eggs, diced onions, bell peppers, zucchini, and your favorite herbs and spices. Pour egg mixture into baking dish and bake for 20-25 minutes, or until eggs are cooked through. Enjoy with a side of fresh fruit.

11. Savory Oatmeal:

Cook oatmeal in water or almond milk. Top with diced tomatoes, cooked spinach, and your favorite herbs and spices. Enjoy with a side of fresh fruit.

12. Sweet Potato Hash:

Heat coconut oil in a skillet over medium heat. Add diced sweet potatoes, onions, bell peppers, and your favorite herbs and spices. Cook until sweet potatoes are tender. Enjoy with a side of fresh fruit.

13. Egg and Vegetable Frittata:

Preheat oven to 350°F. Grease a baking dish with coconut oil. Whisk together eggs, diced onions, bell peppers, zucchini, and your favorite herbs and spices. Pour egg mixture into baking dish and bake for 20-25 minutes, or until eggs are cooked through. Enjoy with a side of fresh fruit.

14. Apple Walnut Oatmeal:

Cook oatmeal in water or almond milk. Top with diced apples, walnuts, and a sprinkle of cinnamon. Enjoy with a side of fresh fruit.

15. Greek Yogurt Bowl:

Top low-fat Greek yogurt with your favorite fresh fruit, nuts, and seeds. Drizzle with honey.

16. Banana Protein Pancakes:

Combine protein powder, almond milk, mashed banana, and egg in a bowl. Heat coconut oil in a skillet over medium heat. Drop spoonfuls of batter onto skillet and cook until pancakes are golden brown. Enjoy with a side of fresh fruit.

17. Vegetable and Egg White Omelet:

Heat coconut oil in a skillet over medium heat. Add diced onions, bell peppers, zucchini, and your favorite herbs and spices. Whisk together egg whites and pour into skillet. Cook until eggs are cooked through. Enjoy with a side of fresh fruit.

18. Egg and Spinach Sandwich:

Spread mashed avocado on toasted whole grain bread. Top with scrambled egg and cooked spinach. Enjoy with a side of fresh fruit.

19. Almond Butter Banana Toast:

Spread almond butter on toasted whole grain bread. Top with sliced banana and a sprinkle of cinnamon.

20. Protein Power Bowl:

Combine cooked quinoa, diced tomatoes, cooked spinach, and your favorite herbs and spices in a bowl. Top with a scoop of your favorite protein powder. Enjoy with a side of fresh fruit.

21. Green Smoothie Bowl:

Blend together spinach, avocado, banana, and almond milk. Pour into a bowl and top with your favorite fresh fruit, nuts, and seeds.

22. PB&J Overnight Oats:

Combine rolled oats, chia seeds, almond milk, and peanut butter in a mason jar. Let sit overnight in the refrigerator, then top with your favorite jelly in the morning.

23. Chia Pudding:

Combine chia seeds, almond milk, and honey in a mason jar. Let sit in the refrigerator for at least an hour, or overnight. Top with your favorite fresh fruit in the morning.

24. Egg, Spinach, and Tomato Breakfast Wrap:

Spread mashed avocado on a whole grain tortilla. Top with scrambled egg, cooked spinach, and diced tomatoes. Roll up and enjoy.

25. Protein Pancakes with Berries:

Combine protein powder, almond milk, mashed banana, and egg in a bowl. Heat coconut oil in a skillet over medium heat. Drop spoonfuls of batter onto skillet and cook until pancakes are golden brown. Top with your favorite berries.

26. Egg and Veggie Breakfast Burrito:

Heat coconut oil in a skillet over medium heat. Add diced onions, bell peppers, zucchini, and your favorite herbs and spices. Whisk together eggs and pour into skillet. Cook until eggs are cooked through. Wrap eggs, vegetables, and a sprinkle of with parchment paper. Press oat mixture into dish and bake at 350°F for 20 minutes. Let cool before slicing into bars. Enjoy with a side of fresh fruit.

27. Overnight Oats with Apple:

Combine rolled oats, chia seeds, almond milk, maple syrup and diced apple in a jar and let it sit overnight.

28. Greek Yogurt and Fruit Bowl:

Top Greek yogurt with your favorite fruits and nuts for a nutritious breakfast.

29. Avocado Egg Toast:

Spread mashed avocado on toasted whole grain bread. Top with poached egg and a sprinkle of sea salt.

30. Chia Seed Pudding with Berries:

Combine chia seeds, almond milk, and honey in a mason jar. Let sit in the refrigerator for at least an hour, or overnight. Top with your favorite berries in the morning.

31. Zucchini Muffins:

Preheat oven to 375°F. Grease a muffin tin with coconut oil. Whisk together eggs, shredded zucchini, and your favorite herbs and spices. Divide egg mixture into muffin tin and bake for 20-25 minutes, or until eggs are cooked through. Enjoy with a side of fresh fruit.

32. Spinach and Feta Egg Muffins:

Preheat oven to 375°F. Grease a muffin tin with coconut oil. Whisk together eggs, cooked spinach, and feta cheese. Divide egg mixture into muffin tin and bake for 20-25 minutes, or until eggs are cooked through. Enjoy with a side of fresh fruit.

33. Oatmeal with Nuts and Fruit:

Cook oatmeal in water or almond milk. Top with your favorite nuts, seeds, and fresh fruit.

34. Broccoli and Cheese Frittata:

Preheat oven to 350°F. Grease a baking dish with coconut oil. Whisk together eggs, shredded broccoli, and shredded cheese. Pour egg mixture into baking dish and bake for 20-25 minutes, or until eggs are cooked through. Enjoy with a side of fresh fruit.

35. Sweet Potato and Egg Hash:

Heat coconut oil in a skillet over medium heat. Add diced sweet potatoes, onions, bell peppers, and your favorite herbs and spices. Whisk together eggs and pour into skillet. Cook until eggs are cooked through. Enjoy with a side of fresh fruit.

36. Protein Waffles:

Combine protein powder, almond milk, mashed banana, and egg in a bowl. Heat waffle iron and drop spoonfuls of batter onto waffle iron. Cook until waffles are golden brown. Enjoy with a side of fresh fruit.

37. Greek Yogurt with Nuts and Fruit:

Top low-fat Greek yogurt with your favorite nuts, seeds, and fresh fruit. Drizzle with honey.

38. Apple Cinnamon Protein Pancakes:

Combine protein powder, almond milk, mashed banana, and egg in a bowl. Heat coconut oil in a skillet over medium heat. Drop spoonfuls of batter onto skillet and cook until pancakes are golden brown. Top with diced apples and a sprinkle of cinnamon.

39. Zucchini Fritters:

Heat coconut oil in a skillet over medium heat. Combine shredded zucchini, eggs, and your favorite herbs and spices. Drop spoonfuls of batter into skillet and cook until fritters are golden brown. Enjoy with a side of fresh fruit.

40. Protein Oatmeal:

Cook oatmeal in water or almond milk. Top with your favorite protein powder and fresh fruit.

41. Baked Egg Cups:

Preheat oven to 350°F. Grease a muffin tin with coconut oil. Whisk together eggs and your favorite herbs and spices. Divide egg mixture into muffin tin and bake for 20-25 minutes, or until eggs are cooked through. Enjoy with a side of fresh fruit.

42. Egg and Veggie Breakfast Bowl:

Heat coconut oil in a skillet over medium heat. Add diced onions, bell peppers, zucchini, and your favorite herbs and spices. Whisk together eggs and pour into skillet. Cook until eggs are cooked through. Serve eggs and vegetables over cooked quinoa and top with a sprinkle of your favorite cheese.

43. Almond Butter Overnight Oats:

Combine rolled oats, chia seeds, almond milk, and almond butter in a mason jar. Let sit overnight in the refrigerator, then top with your favorite fresh fruit in the morning.

44. Avocado Toast with Egg:

Spread mashed avocado on toasted whole grain bread and top with poached egg.

45. Baked Apple:

Preheat oven to 350°F. Grease a baking dish with coconut oil. Place an apple in the baking dish and fill the center with a mixture of nuts, seeds, and honey. Bake for 20-25 minutes, or until apples are tender. Enjoy with a side of fresh fruit.

46. Kale and Feta Egg Muffins:

Preheat oven to 375°F. Grease a muffin tin with coconut oil. Whisk together eggs, cooked kale, and feta cheese. Divide egg mixture into muffin tin and bake for 20-25 minutes, or until eggs are cooked through. Enjoy with a side of fresh fruit.

47. Quinoa Breakfast Bowl:

Cook quinoa in water or almond milk. Top with diced tomatoes, cooked spinach, and your favorite herbs and spices. Enjoy with a side of fresh fruit.

48. Smoothie Bowl:

Blend together your favorite fruits and vegetables with almond milk. Pour into a bowl and top with your favorite nuts, seeds, and fresh fruit.

49. Egg and Avocado Breakfast Sandwich:

Spread mashed avocado on toasted whole grain bread. Top with poached egg and your favorite herbs and spices.

50. Protein French Toast:

Combine protein powder, almond milk, and egg in a shallow dish. Dip slices of whole grain bread into mixture. Heat coconut oil in a skillet over medium heat and cook bread until golden brown. Enjoy with a side of fresh fruit.

51. Baked Sweet Potato:

Preheat oven to 375°F. Grease a baking dish with coconut oil. Pierce a sweet potato with a fork and place in baking dish. Bake for 45-60 minutes, or until sweet potato is tender. Top with your favorite nuts, seeds, and fresh fruit.

52. Omelet with Veggies:

Heat coconut oil in a skillet over medium heat. Add diced onions, bell peppers, zucchini, and your favorite herbs and spices. Whisk together eggs and pour into skillet. Cook until eggs are cooked through. Enjoy with a side of fresh fruit.

53. Egg and Veggie Breakfast Pizza:

Preheat oven to 375°F. Grease a baking dish with coconut oil. Spread mashed avocado on a whole grain tortilla. Top with scrambled eggs, cooked vegetables, and your favorite herbs and spices. Bake for 10-15 minutes, or until eggs are cooked through. Enjoy with a side of fresh fruit.

54. Banana Oat Greek Yogurt:

Layer low-fat Greek yogurt, mashed banana, and your favorite granola in a bowl. Drizzle with honey.

55. Carrot Cake Overnight Oats:

Combine rolled oats, chia seeds, almond milk, shredded carrots, and a sprinkle of cinnamon in a mason jar. Let sit overnight in the refrigerator, then top with your favorite nuts and seeds in the morning.

56. Protein Toast:

Spread your favorite nut butter on toasted whole grain bread. Top with a scoop of your favorite protein powder.

57. Sweet Potato Hash with Eggs:

Heat coconut oil in a skillet over medium heat. Add diced sweet potatoes, onions, bell peppers, and your favorite herbs and spices. Whisk together eggs and pour into skillet. Cook until eggs are cooked through. Enjoy with a side of fresh fruit.

58. Green Smoothie:

Blend together spinach, avocado, banana, and almond milk. Enjoy with a sprinkle of chia seeds and cinnamon.

59. Baked Oatmeal:

Preheat oven to 350°F. Grease a baking dish with coconut oil. Combine rolled oats, chia seeds, almond milk, diced apples, and a sprinkle of cinnamon in a bowl. Pour oat mixture into baking dish and bake for 20 minutes. Let cool before slicing into bars. Enjoy with a side of fresh fruit.

60. Protein Pancakes with Nuts and Fruit:

Combine protein powder, almond milk, mashed banana, and egg in a bowl. Heat coconut oil in a skillet over medium heat. Drop spoonfuls of batter onto skillet and cook until pancakes are golden brown. Top with your favorite nuts, seeds, and fresh fruit.

61. Egg Muffins with Veggies:

Preheat oven to 375°F. Grease a muffin tin with coconut oil. Whisk together eggs, diced onions, bell peppers, zucchini, and your favorite herbs and spices. Divide egg mixture into muffin tin and bake for 20-25 minutes, or until eggs are cooked through. Enjoy with a side of fresh fruit.

62. Blueberry Protein Pancakes:

Combine protein powder, almond milk, mashed banana, and egg in a bowl. Heat coconut oil in a skillet over medium heat. Drop spoonfuls of batter onto skillet and cook until pancakes are golden brown. Top with your favorite blueberries.

63. Oatmeal Breakfast Bars:

Preheat oven to 350°F. Grease a baking dish with coconut oil. Combine rolled oats, chia seeds, almond milk, diced apples, and a sprinkle of cinnamon in a bowl. Press oat mixture into dish and bake for 20 minutes. Let cool before slicing into bars. Enjoy with a side of fresh fruit.

64. Vegetable Omelet:

Heat coconut oil in a skillet over medium heat. Add diced onions, bell peppers, zucchini, and your favorite herbs and spices. Whisk together eggs and pour into skillet. Cook until eggs are cooked through. Enjoy with a side of fresh fruit.

65. Baked Egg Cups with Vegetables:

Preheat oven to 350°F. Grease a muffin tin with coconut oil. Whisk together eggs, diced onions, bell peppers, zucchini, and your favorite herbs and spices. Divide egg mixture into muffin tin and bake for 20-25 minutes, or until eggs are cooked through. Enjoy with a side of fresh fruit.

66. Peanut Butter Banana Smoothie:

Blend together 1 banana, 1 tablespoon of peanut butter, and ¾ cup of almond milk. Enjoy with a sprinkle of chia seeds and cinnamon.

67. Sweet Potato Toast with Avocado:

Spread mashed sweet potato on toasted whole grain bread. Top with mashed avocado and a sprinkle of sea salt.

68. Zucchini Fritters with Avocado:

Heat coconut oil in a skillet over medium heat. Combine shredded zucchini, eggs, and your favorite herbs and spices. Drop spoonfuls of batter into skillet and cook until fritters are golden brown. Top with mashed avocado and a sprinkle of sea salt.

69. Apple Pie Oatmeal:

Cook oatmeal in water or almond milk. Top with diced apples, walnuts, and a sprinkle of cinnamon.

70. Egg, Spinach, and Tomato Breakfast Bowl:

Heat coconut oil in a skillet over medium heat. Add diced onions, bell peppers, zucchini, and your favorite herbs and spices. Whisk together eggs and pour into skillet. Cook until eggs are cooked through. Serve eggs and vegetables over cooked quinoa and top with diced tomatoes and cooked spinach.

71. Baked Apples with Nuts and Seeds:

Preheat oven to 350°F. Grease a baking dish with coconut oil. Place an apple in the baking dish and fill the center with a mixture of your favorite nuts and seeds. Bake for 20-25 minutes, or until apples are tender. Enjoy with a side of fresh fruit.

72. Sweet Potato Toast with Egg:

Spread mashed sweet potato on toasted whole grain bread. Top with poached egg and a sprinkle of sea salt.

73. Blue Smoothie Bowl:

Blend together your favorite blueberries, banana, and almond milk. Pour into a bowl and top with your favorite nuts, seeds, and fresh fruit.

74. Banana Walnut Protein Pancakes:

Combine protein powder, almond milk, mashed banana, and egg in a bowl. Heat coconut oil in a skillet over medium heat. Drop spoonfuls of batter onto skillet and cook until pancakes are golden brown. Top with your favorite walnuts.

75. Egg and Veggie Breakfast Wrap:

Heat coco81. Strawberry Protein Pancakes: Combine protein powder, almond milk, mashed banana, and egg in a bowl. Heat coconut oil in a skillet over medium heat. Drop spoonful of batter onto skillet and cook until pancakes are golden brown. Top with your favorite strawberries nut oil in a skillet over medium heat. Add diced onions, bell peppers, zucchini, and your favorite herbs and spices. Whisk together eggs and pour into skillet. Cook until eggs are cooked through.

Wrap eggs, vegetables, and a sprinkle of cheese in a whole grain tortilla. Enjoy with a side of fresh fruit.

76. Quinoa Porridge:

Cook quinoa in water or almond milk. Top with diced apples, walnuts, and a sprinkle of cinnamon.

77. Avocado Toast with Tomatoes:

Spread mashed avocado on toasted whole grain bread and top with diced tomatoes and a sprinkle of sea salt.

78. Kale and Feta Egg Cups:

Preheat oven to 375 °F. Grease a muffin tin with coconut oil. Whisk together eggs, cooked kale, and feta cheese. Divide egg mixture into muffin tin and bake for 20-25 minutes, or until eggs are cooked through. Enjoy with a side of fresh fruit.

79. Apple Cinnamon Oatmeal:

Cook oatmeal in water or almond milk. Top with diced apples and a sprinkle of cinnamon.

80. Mashed Sweet Potato Toast:

Spread mashed sweet potato on toasted whole grain bread. Top with your favorite nuts, seeds, and fresh fruit.

81. Strawberry Protein Pancakes:

Combine protein powder, almond milk, mashed banana,

and egg in a bowl. Heat coconut oil in a skillet over medium heat. Drop spoonful of batter onto skillet and cook until pancakes are golden brown. Top with your favorite strawberries

82. Broccoli and Cheese Frittata:

Preheat oven to 350°F. Grease a baking dish with coconut oil. Whisk together eggs, shredded broccoli, and shredded cheese. Pour egg mixture into baking dish and bake for 20-25 minutes, or until eggs are cooked through. Enjoy with a side of fresh fruit.

83. Banana Nut Butter Smoothie:

Blend together 1 banana, 1 tablespoon of nut butter, and ¾ cup of almond milk. Enjoy with a sprinkle of chia seeds and cinnamon.

84. Oatmeal with Nuts and Seeds:

Cook oatmeal in water or almond milk. Top with your favorite nuts, seeds, and fresh fruit.

85. Blueberry Overnight Oats:

Combine rolled oats, chia seeds, almond milk, and your favorite blueberries in a mason jar. Let sit overnight in the refrigerator, then top with your favorite nuts and seeds in the morning.

86. Avocado Toast with Egg and Spinach:

Spread mashed avocado on toasted whole grain bread and top with poached egg and cooked spinach.

87. Zucchini Bread:

Preheat oven to 375°F. Grease a baking dish with coconut oil. Whisk together eggs, shredded zucchini, and your favorite herbs and spices. Pour egg mixture into baking dish and bake for 20-25 minutes, or until eggs are cooked through. Enjoy with a side of fresh fruit.

88. Egg and Veggie Breakfast Burrito Bowl:

Heat coconut oil in a skillet over medium heat. Add diced onions, bell peppers, zucchini, and your favorite herbs and spices. Whisk together eggs and pour into skillet. Cook until eggs are cooked through. Serve eggs and vegetables over cooked quinoa and top with a sprinkle of cheese.

89. Protein French toast with Berries:

Combine protein powder, almond milk, and egg in a shallow dish. Dip slices of whole grain bread into mixture. Heat coconut oil in a skillet over medium heat and cook bread until golden brown. Top with your favorite berries.

90. Apple Pie Smoothie

Blend together diced apples, banana, almond milk, and a sprinkle of cinnamon. Enjoy with a sprinkle of chia seeds.

91. Egg and Avocado Breakfast Sandwich:

Spread mashed avocado on toasted whole grain bread and top with poached egg and your favorite herbs and spices.

92. Spinach and Feta Egg Cups:

Preheat oven to 375°F. Grease a muffin tin with coconut oil. Whisk together eggs, cooked spinach, and feta cheese. Divide egg mixture into muffin tin and bake for 20-25 minutes, or until eggs are cooked through. Enjoy with a side of fresh fruit.

93. Quinoa Breakfast Burrito:

Cook quinoa in water or almond milk. Top with diced onions, bell peppers, zucchini, and your favorite herbs and spices. Wrap quinoa and vegetables in a whole grain tortilla. Enjoy with a side of fresh fruit.

94. Baked Sweet Potato with Nuts and Seeds:

Preheat oven to 375°F. Grease a baking dish with coconut oil. Pierce a sweet potato with a fork and place in baking dish. Bake for 45-60 minutes, or until sweet potato is tender. Top with your favorite nuts, seeds, and fresh fruit.

95. Protein Oatmeal with Berries:

Cook oatmeal in water or almond milk. Top with your favorite protein powder and fresh fruit.

96. Avocado Egg Toast with Spinach:

Spread mashed avocado on toasted whole grain bread. Top with poached egg, cooked spinach, and a sprinkle of sea salt.

97. Egg and Veggie Breakfast Sandwich:

Heat coconut oil in a skillet over medium heat. Add diced onions, bell peppers, zucchini, and your favorite herbs and spices. Whisk together eggs and pour into skillet. Cook until eggs are cooked through. Place eggs and vegetables on toasted whole grain bread and top with a sprinkle of cheese. Enjoy with a side of fresh fruit.

98. Blueberry Coconut Oatmeal:

Cook oatmeal in water or almond milk. Top with your favorite blueberries and a sprinkle of coconut flakes.

99. Kale and Feta Egg Wrap:

Heat coconut oil in a skillet over medium heat. Add cooked kale and feta cheese. Whisk together eggs and pour into skillet. Cook until eggs are cooked through. Wrap eggs, kale, and feta in a whole grain tortilla. Enjoy with a side of fresh fruit.

100. Protein Waffles with Nuts and Fruit:

Combine protein powder, almond milk, mashed banana, and egg in a bowl. Heat a waffle iron and cook until golden brown. Top with your favorite nuts, seeds, and fresh fruit.

LUNCH

101. Roasted Vegetable Wrap:

Spread hummus on a whole-wheat wrap, and layer on roasted vegetables like bell peppers, onions, and mushrooms, along with spinach and feta cheese.

102. Quinoa Bowl:

Top cooked quinoa with grilled chicken, roasted sweet potatoes, and sautéed spinach.

103. Mediterranean Salad:

Toss together romaine lettuce, chickpeas, olives, diced tomatoes, cucumbers, and feta cheese. Drizzle with a light vinaigrette.

104. Deli Roll-Ups:

Spread a whole-wheat wrap with mustard or hummus, and top with sliced deli turkey, avocado, and spinach. Roll up and enjoy.

105. Wild Salmon Salad:

Toss together cooked wild salmon, roasted sweet potatoes, cucumbers, tomatoes, and crumbled feta cheese. Drizzle with a light lemon-dill dressing.

106. Turkey Sandwich:

Spread a whole-grain roll with a thin layer of mayonnaise, and top with sliced turkey, lettuce, and tomato.

107. Peanut Butter and Banana Sandwich:

Spread peanut butter on whole-grain bread, and top with banana slices.

108. Baked Egg Wrap:

Spread a whole-wheat wrap with hummus, top with egg slices and shredded cheese, and bake until cheese is melted.

109. Veggie Burger:

Grill a veggie burger and top with lettuce, tomato, and a light Greek yogurt sauce.

110. Zucchini Noodles:

Toss zucchini noodles with grilled chicken, roasted peppers, and tomatoes.

111. Avocado Toast:

Toast a slice of whole-grain bread and top with mashed avocado and a sprinkle of red pepper flakes.

112. Tuna Salad:

Mix together canned tuna, diced celery, and light mayonnaise. Serve over a bed of lettuce.

113. Spinach Salad:

Toss together baby spinach, diced apples, walnuts, and crumbled feta cheese. Drizzle with a light balsamic dressing.

114. Mexican Rice Bowl:

Top cooked brown rice with grilled vegetables, black beans, and salsa.

115. Cucumber Sandwich:

Spread whole-wheat bread with light mayonnaise, and top with cucumber slices and feta cheese.

116. Lentil Soup:

Simmer lentils with onions, carrots, and broth.

117. Turkey and Veggie Skewers:

Thread turkey cubes and vegetables onto skewers, and grill until cooked through.

118. Quinoa Stuffed Peppers:

Fill bell peppers with cooked quinoa, diced tomatoes, and feta cheese.

119. Curried Chicken Salad:

Mix together diced chicken, celery, red onion, and raisins. Drizzle with a light curry dressing.

120. Cobb Salad:

Toss together lettuce, diced turkey, crumbled bacon, boiled egg, avocado, and blue cheese.

121. Kale and Quinoa Bowl:

Top cooked quinoa with kale, roasted vegetables, and grilled chicken.

122. Asian Noodle Bowl:

Top cooked soba noodles with grilled shrimp, bok choy, mushrooms, and carrots. Drizzle with a light teriyaki sauce.

123. Egg Salad:

Mix together boiled eggs, diced celery, and light mayonnaise. Serve on top of a bed of lettuce.

124. Hummus and Veggie Wrap:

Spread a whole-wheat wrap with hummus, and top with cucumbers, bell peppers, tomatoes, and spinach.

125. Greek Salad:

Toss together lettuce, olives, feta cheese, cucumbers, tomatoes, and diced chicken. Drizzle with a light vinaigrette.

126. Tuna Melt:

Spread a whole-wheat wrap with light mayonnaise, top with canned tuna, and sprinkle with shredded cheese. Bake in the oven until cheese is melted.

127. Avocado Egg Salad:

Mash together boiled eggs and avocado, and season with salt and pepper. Serve on top of whole-grain toast.

128. Mediterranean Chicken Wrap:

Spread a whole-wheat wrap with hummus, top with grilled chicken, cucumber, tomatoes, and feta cheese.

129. Broccoli and Cheese Omelet:

Sauté broccoli in a pan, and pour over beaten eggs. Sprinkle with shredded cheese and bake until eggs are cooked through.

130. Turkey and Veggie Sandwich:

Spread whole-grain bread with light mayonnaise, and top with sliced turkey, lettuce, and tomato.

131. Lentil and Vegetable Soup:

Simmer lentils with onions, carrots, celery, and vegetable broth.

132. Baked Sweet Potato:

Pierce a sweet potato with a fork and bake in the oven until tender. Top with Greek yogurt, diced tomatoes, and feta cheese.

133. Quinoa and Veggie Salad:

Toss together cooked quinoa, diced vegetables, and sunflower seeds. Drizzle with a light vinaigrette.

134. Egg and Avocado Toast:

Toast a slice of whole-grain bread and top with mashed avocado and a boiled egg.

135. Turkey and Quinoa Bowl:

Top cooked quinoa with grilled turkey, roasted vegetables, and feta cheese.

136. Fruit Salad:

Toss together diced pineapple, strawberries, and apples. Drizzle with a light honey-lemon dressing.

137. Vegetable Soup:

Simmer carrots, onions, celery, and potatoes in vegetable broth.

138. Bacon, Spinach, and Cheese Wrap:

Spread a whole-wheat wrap with light mayonnaise, and top with cooked bacon, spinach, and shredded cheese.

139. Falafel Wrap:

Top a whole-wheat wrap with falafel, lettuce, tomatoes, and light tzatziki sauce.

140. Greek Yogurt Parfait:

Layer Greek yogurt with fresh fruit and a sprinkle of walnuts.

141. Chicken Salad Sandwich:

Mix together cooked chicken, celery, and light mayonnaise. Serve on top of whole-grain toast.

142. Quinoa and Black Bean Burrito:

Spread a whole-wheat wrap with refried beans, and top with cooked quinoa, black beans, and diced vegetables.

143. Tuna and Avocado Salad:

Mix together canned tuna, diced avocado, and a light vinaigrette. Serve on top of a bed of lettuce.

144. Grilled Vegetables:

Grill a variety of vegetables like bell peppers, onions, mushrooms, and zucchini.

145. Roasted Eggplant Sandwich:

Spread a whole-grain roll with light mayonnaise, and top with roasted eggplant slices and feta cheese.

146. Egg and Vegetable Frittata:

Sauté vegetables in a pan, pour over beaten eggs, and sprinkle with shredded cheese. Bake until eggs are cooked through.

147. Chickpea Salad:

Mix together chickpeas, diced celery, and light mayonnaise. Serve on top of whole-grain toast.

148. Chicken and Rice Bowl:

Top cooked brown rice with grilled chicken, roasted vegetables, and diced tomatoes.

149. Avocado and Egg Toast:

Toast a slice of whole-grain bread and top with mashed avocado and a boiled egg.

150. Mango Smoothie:

Blend together frozen mango, Greek yogurt, and a splash of almond milk.

151. Tomato and Mozzarella Sandwich: Layer mozzarella cheese and tomato slices onto whole-grain bread, and top with a sprinkle of oregano.

152. Hummus and Veggie Sandwich:

Spread whole-grain bread with hummus, and top with cucumbers, bell peppers, tomatoes, and spinach.

153. Curry Bowl:

Top cooked brown rice with cooked vegetables, chickpeas, and a light curry sauce.

154. Tofu and Veggie Stir-Fry:

Sauté vegetables in a pan, and add in cubed tofu.

155. Salmon and Rice Bowl:

Top cooked brown rice with grilled salmon, roasted vegetables, and a light soy sauce.

156. Zucchini Fritters:

Mix together grated zucchini, beaten eggs, and a sprinkle of parmesan cheese. Fry in a pan until golden brown.

157. Egg and Cheese Sandwich:

Spread a whole-grain roll with light mayonnaise, and top with a fried egg and shredded cheese.

158. Fruit Salad Bowl:

Mix together diced pineapple, strawberries, and apples. Top with Greek yogurt and a sprinkle of almonds.

159. Turkey and Cheese Sandwich:

Spread a whole-grain roll with light mayonnaise, and top with sliced turkey and shredded cheese.

160. Lentil Salad:

Toss together cooked lentils, diced vegetables, and a light vinaigrette.

161. Baked Potato:

Pierce a potato with a fork and bake in the oven until tender. Top with Greek yogurt, diced tomatoes, and feta cheese.

162. Egg and Avocado Wrap:

Spread a whole-wheat wrap with light mayonnaise, and top with a fried egg and mashed avocado.

163. Veggie Omelet:

Sauté vegetables in a pan, pour over beaten eggs, and bake until eggs are cooked through.

164. Quinoa-Stuffed Peppers:

Fill bell peppers with cooked quinoa, diced tomatoes, and feta cheese.

165. Greek Salad Bowl:

Top cooked brown rice with lettuce, olives, feta cheese, cucumbers, tomatoes, and diced chicken. Drizzle with a light vinaigrette.

166. BBQ Chicken Sandwich:

Spread a whole-grain roll with BBQ sauce, and top with sliced chicken and coleslaw.

167. Chickpea and Vegetable Wrap:

Spread a whole-wheat wrap with hummus, and top with chickpeas, roasted vegetables, and feta cheese.

168. Tomato Soup:

Simmer tomatoes, onions, and vegetable broth in a pot.

169. Roasted Vegetable Sandwich:

Spread a whole-grain roll with light mayonnaise, and top with roasted vegetables, feta cheese, and spinach.

170. Fruit and Yogurt Bowl:

Layer Greek yogurt with fresh fruit and a sprinkle of almonds.

171. Egg Salad Wrap:

Spread a whole-wheat wrap with light mayonnaise, and top with boiled eggs and diced celery.

172. Turkey and Cheese Wrap:

Spread a whole-wheat wrap with light mayonnaise, and top with sliced turkey and shredded cheese.

173. Lentil and Rice Bowl:

Top cooked brown rice with cooked lentils, diced vegetables, and light vinaigrette.

174. Quinoa and Black Bean Salad:

Toss together cooked quinoa, black beans, diced vegetables, and light vinaigrette.

175. Vegetable and Cheese Omelet:

Sauté vegetables in a pan, pour over beaten eggs, and sprinkle with shredded cheese. Bake until eggs are cooked through.

176. Baked Sweet Potato and Bean Burrito:

Spread a whole-wheat wrap with refried beans, and top with a baked sweet potato and black beans.

177. Turkey Burger:

Grill a turkey burger and top with lettuce, tomato, and a light Greek yogurt sauce.

178. Mediterranean Quinoa Bowl:

Top cooked quinoa with grilled chicken, roasted vegetables, and feta cheese.

179. Grilled Cheese Sandwich:

Spread a whole-grain roll with light mayonnaise, and top with shredded cheese.

180. Greek Yogurt Parfait:

Layer Greek yogurt with fresh fruit and a sprinkle of almonds.

181. Baked Potato and Egg:

Pierce a potato with a fork and bake in the oven until tender. Top with a fried egg and shredded cheese.

182. Tofu Scramble:

Sauté cubed tofu in a pan, and scramble with beaten eggs.

183. Hummus and Veggie Toast:

Toast a slice of whole-grain bread and top with hummus and diced vegetables.

184. Egg and Vegetable Frittata:

Sauté vegetables in a pan, pour over beaten eggs, and sprinkle with shredded cheese. Bake until eggs are cooked through.

185. Chicken and Rice Soup:

Simmer cooked chicken, rice, and vegetable broth in a pot.

186. Curry Bowl:

Top cooked brown rice with cooked vegetables, chickpeas, and a light curry sauce.

187. Tuna and Avocado Wrap:

Spread a whole-wheat wrap with light mayonnaise, and top with canned tuna, diced avocado, and lettuce.

188. Quinoa and Vegetable Salad:

Toss together cooked quinoa, diced vegetables, and sunflower seeds. Drizzle with a light vinaigrette.

189. Turkey and Veggie Sandwich:

Spread whole-grain bread with light mayonnaise, and top with sliced turkey, lettuce, and tomato.

190. Egg and Cheese Wrap:

Spread a whole-wheat wrap with light mayonnaise, and top with a fried egg and shredded cheese.

191. Baked Eggplant Sandwich:

Spread a whole-grain roll with light mayonnaise, and top with roasted eggplant slices and feta cheese.

192. Lentil Soup:

Simmer lentils with onions, carrots, and vegetable broth.

193. Mango Smoothie:

Blend together frozen mango, Greek yogurt, and a splash of almond milk.

194. Falafel Wrap:

Top a whole-wheat wrap with falafel, lettuce, tomatoes, and light tzatziki sauce.

195. Chickpea Salad:

Mix together chickpeas, diced celery, and light mayonnaise. Serve on top of whole-grain toast.

196. Baked Potato and Bean Burrito:

Spread a whole-wheat wrap with refried beans, and top with a baked potato and black beans.

197. Vegetable Soup:

Simmer carrots, onions, celery, and potatoes in vegetable broth.

198. Tofu and Veggie Stir-Fry:

Sauté vegetables in a pan, and add in cubed tofu.

199. Avocado Toast:

Toast a slice of whole-grain bread and top with mashed avocado and a sprinkle of red pepper flakes.

200. Curried Chicken Salad:

Mix together diced chicken, celery, red onion, and raisins. Drizzle with a light curry dressing.

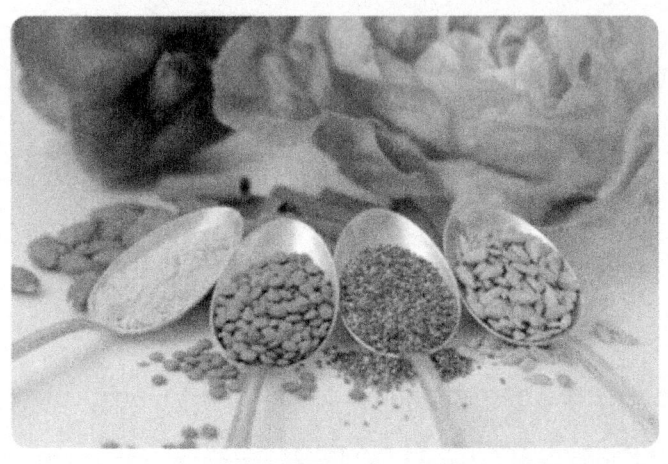

DINNER

201. Mediterranean Quinoa Bowl:

Cook quinoa according to package instructions, top with olive oil, diced tomatoes, feta cheese, black olives and parsley.

202. Veggie Stir Fry:

Heat olive oil in a skillet, add diced onion, bell peppers, mushrooms, and garlic. Cook for 5 minutes. Add in cooked quinoa, diced carrots, chopped broccoli and a dash of soy sauce. Cook for another 5 minutes.

203. Grilled Chicken Salad:

Grill 2 chicken breasts. Cut into cubes and place on a bed of spinach and Romaine lettuce. Top with sliced avocado, diced tomatoes and light vinaigrette.

204. Turkey and Veggie Burgers:

Combine ground turkey, diced onion, bell peppers, garlic and spices in a bowl. Form into patties and grill. Serve on whole grain buns with lettuce and tomato.

205. Roasted Veggie and Quinoa Bowl: Preheat oven to 400°F. Toss cubed sweet potatoes, zucchini, bell peppers, onion and garlic with olive oil and salt. Roast for 25 minutes. Serve over cooked quinoa and top with crumbled feta cheese.

206. Grilled Salmon with Asparagus: Grill 2 salmon fillets and 4 spears of asparagus. Serve with a lemon garlic sauce.

207. Baked Tilapia with Sweet Potato: Preheat oven to 400°F. Place 2 tilapia fillets on a baking sheet. Top with diced sweet potatoes, olive oil, salt and pepper. Bake for 25 minutes.

208. Eggplant Parmesan: Cut 2 eggplants into thin slices. Dip in egg whites, then in bread crumbs. Bake at 350°F for 25 minutes. Top with marinara sauce and mozzarella cheese. Bake for an additional 10 minutes.

209. Turkey Chili:

Cook 1 pound of ground turkey in a large pot. Add diced onion, bell peppers, garlic, chili powder, cumin, oregano, and tomato sauce. Simmer for 20 minutes.

210. Zucchini Noodles with Avocado Pesto:

Spiralize 2 zucchinis. Toss with avocado pesto (made of avocado, garlic, basil, pine nuts, olive oil, and lemon juice). Top with diced tomatoes and feta cheese.

211. Baked Tilapia with Roasted Tomatoes:

Preheat oven to 450°F. Place 2 tilapia fillets on a baking sheet. Top with diced tomatoes, olive oil, salt and pepper. Bake for 20 minutes.

212. Turkey Taco Salad:

Heat olive oil in a skillet and cook 1 pound of ground turkey. Add taco seasoning, diced onion, bell peppers, and garlic. Serve in a bowl of lettuce with diced tomatoes, black beans, avocado and a light vinaigrette.

213. Baked Salmon with Broccoli:

Preheat oven to 425°F. Place 2 salmon fillets on a baking sheet. Top with diced broccoli, olive oil, salt and pepper. Bake for 20 minutes.

214. Quinoa Salad:

Cook quinoa according to package instructions. Toss with diced cucumber, feta cheese, black olives, diced tomatoes, and a light vinaigrette.

215. Baked Eggplant Parmesan:

Cut 2 eggplants into thin slices. Dip in egg whites, then in bread crumbs. Bake at 350°F for 25 minutes. Top with marinara sauce and mozzarella cheese. Bake for an additional 10 minutes.

216. Grilled Vegetable Skewers:

Heat a grill to medium-high heat. Thread bell peppers, zucchini, mushrooms, and onion onto skewers. Grill for 8 minutes, turning occasionally.

217. Turkey and Veggie Stuffed Peppers:

Cut the tops off of 4 bell peppers. Remove the seeds. In a large bowl, combine 1 pound of ground turkey with diced onion, bell peppers, garlic, and spices. Stuff the peppers with the turkey mixture and bake at 350°F for 40 minutes.

218. Roasted Potato and Chickpea Salad:

Preheat oven to 400°F. Toss cubed potatoes, chickpeas, onion, bell pepper, garlic and olive oil. Roast for 25 minutes. Serve over a bed of lettuce and top with diced tomatoes and light vinaigrette.

219. Baked Fish with Spinach:

Preheat oven to 425°F. Place 2 white fish fillets on a baking sheet. Top with spinach, olive oil, salt and pepper. Bake for 20 minutes.

220. Sweet Potato Fries:

Preheat oven to 400°F. Cut 2 sweet potatoes into wedges. Toss with olive oil, salt and pepper. Bake for 25 minutes, flipping once.

221. Grilled Halibut with Mango Salsa: Grill 2 halibut fillets. Serve with a mango salsa (made of diced mango, diced onion, diced bell peppers, lime juice, and cilantro).

222. Quinoa Veggie Burgers: Combine cooked quinoa, diced onion, bell peppers, garlic and spices in a bowl. Form into patties and grill. Serve on whole grain buns with lettuce and tomato.

223. Baked Cod with Roasted Broccoli: Preheat oven to 425°F. Place 2 cod fillets on a baking sheet. Top with diced broccoli, olive oil, salt and pepper. Bake for 20 minutes.

224. Baked Tofu with Asparagus: Preheat oven to 400°F. Cut 1 package of extra firm tofu into cubes. Place on a baking sheet. Top with asparagus, olive oil, salt and pepper. Bake for 25 minutes.

225. Lentil Soup:

Heat olive oil in a large pot. Add diced onion, bell peppers, garlic, and spices. Cook for 5 minutes. Add lentils, vegetable broth, and diced tomatoes. Simmer for 30 minutes.

226. Grilled Chicken with Roasted Vegetables:

Grill 2 chicken breasts. Serve with a side of roasted vegetables (made of cubed sweet potatoes, zucchini, bell peppers, onion, garlic and olive oil).

227. Baked Eggplant and Quinoa Casserole:

Preheat oven to 375°F. Combine cooked quinoa, diced eggplant, diced tomatoes, garlic, and spices in a bowl. Place in a baking dish and top with crumbled feta cheese. Bake for 25 minutes.

228. Turkey and Kale Stuffed Sweet Potatoes:

Preheat oven to 400°F. Bake 4 sweet potatoes for 40 minutes. Meanwhile, heat olive oil in a skillet and cook 1 pound of ground turkey. Add kale and cook for 5 minutes.

Cut the potatoes in half, top with the turkey and kale mixture and serve.

229. Grilled Zucchini Boats:

Cut 2 zucchinis lengthwise. Scoop out the insides. Heat olive oil in a skillet and cook diced onion, bell peppers, garlic, and spices. Fill the zucchinis with the mixture and grill for 10 minutes.

230. Baked Salmon with Spaghetti Squash:

Preheat oven to 425°F. Place 2 salmon fillets on a baking sheet. Top with spaghetti squash, olive oil, salt and pepper. Bake for 20 minutes.

231. Zucchini Lasagna:

Preheat oven to 375°F. Cut 2 zucchinis into thin slices. Layer in a baking dish with marinara sauce, cooked lentils, diced onion, bell peppers, garlic and mozzarella cheese. Bake for 25 minutes.

232. Eggplant and Quinoa Stuffed Peppers:

Cut the tops off of 4 bell peppers. Remove the seeds. In a large bowl, combine cooked quinoa, diced eggplant, garlic, and spices. Stuff the peppers with the mixture and bake at 350°F for 40 minutes.

233. Grilled Portobello Mushrooms:

Heat a grill to medium-high heat. Grill 4 portobello mushrooms for 8 minutes, flipping once. Serve with a side of roasted vegetables.

234. Baked Tilapia with Roasted Asparagus:

Preheat oven to 450°F. Place 2 tilapia fillets on a baking sheet. Top with asparagus, olive oil, salt and pepper. Bake for 20 minutes.

235. Salad Niçoise:

Place a bed of lettuce in a bowl. Top with cooked green beans, diced tomatoes, boiled eggs, tuna, and olives. Drizzle with light vinaigrette.

236. Veggie Fajitas:

Heat olive oil in a skillet. Add diced onion, bell peppers, mushrooms, and garlic. Cook for 5 minutes. Serve in a warm tortilla with diced tomatoes and avocado.

237. Baked Sweet Potato Fries:

Preheat oven to 400°F. Cut 2 sweet potatoes into wedges. Toss with olive oil, salt and pepper. Bake for 25 minutes, flipping once.

238. Grilled Salmon with Spinach:

Grill 2 salmon fillets and a side of spinach. Serve with a lemon garlic sauce.

239. Baked Tofu with Quinoa:

Preheat oven to 400°F. Cut 1 package of extra firm tofu into cubes. Place on a baking sheet. Top with cooked quinoa, olive oil, salt and pepper. Bake for 25 minutes.

240. Roasted Vegetable Soup:

Preheat oven to 400°F. Toss cubed sweet potatoes, zucchini, bell peppers, onion and garlic with olive oil and salt. Roast for 25 minutes. Place the roasted vegetables in a pot and add vegetable broth. Simmer for 20 minutes.

241. Lentil Tacos:

Heat olive oil in a skillet and cook 1 cup of cooked lentils. Add taco seasoning, diced onion, bell peppers, and garlic. Serve in a warm tortilla with diced tomatoes, lettuce and avocado.

242. Turkey and Quinoa Sliders:

Combine ground turkey, cooked quinoa, diced onion, bell peppers, garlic and spices in a bowl. Form into small patties and grill. Serve on whole grain buns with lettuce and tomato.

243. Baked Eggplant Parmesan:

Cut 2 eggplants into thin slices. Dip in egg whites, then in bread crumbs. Bake at 350°F for 25 minutes. Top with marinara sauce and mozzarella cheese. Bake for an additional 10 minutes.

244. Vegetable Curry:

Heat olive oil in a large pot. Add diced onion, bell peppers, garlic, and spices. Cook for 5 minutes. Add diced tomatoes, vegetable broth, and cooked quinoa. Simmer for 20 minutes.

245. Grilled Halibut with Mango Salsa:

Grill 2 halibut fillets. Serve with a mango salsa (made of

diced mango, diced onion, diced bell peppers, lime juice, and cilantro).

246. Stuffed Zucchini:

Preheat oven to 350°F. Cut 2 zucchinis in half lengthwise. Scoop out the insides. Heat olive oil in a skillet and cook diced onion, bell peppers, garlic, and spices. Fill the zucchinis with the mixture and bake for 25 minutes.

247. Cauliflower Rice Bowl:

Heat olive oil in a skillet. Add diced onion, bell peppers, garlic, and spices. Cook for 5 minutes. Add riced cauliflower and cook for an additional 5 minutes. Serve with diced tomatoes, black beans, and light vinaigrette.

248. Baked Tilapia with Broccoli:

Preheat oven to 450°F. Place 2 tilapia fillets on a baking sheet. Top with diced broccoli, olive oil, salt and pepper. Bake for 20 minutes.

249. Baked Eggplant with Quinoa:

Preheat oven to 375°F. Cut 2 eggplants into cubes. Place on a baking sheet. Top with cooked quinoa, olive oil, salt and pepper. Bake for 25 minutes.

250. Grilled Shrimp with Roasted Vegetables:

Heat a grill to medium-high heat Grill 4 shrimp for 4 minutes, flipping once. Serve with a side of roasted vegetables (made of cubed sweet potatoes, zucchini, bell peppers, onion, garlic and olive).

251. Baked Sweet Potato Fries:

Preheat oven to 400°F. Cut 2 sweet potatoes into wedges. Toss with olive oil, salt and pepper. Bake for 25 minutes, flipping once.

252. Eggplant and Lentil Curry:

Heat olive oil in a large pot. Add diced eggplant, onion, bell peppers, garlic, and spices. Cook for 5 minutes. Add lentils, diced tomatoes, and vegetable broth. Simmer for 20 minutes.

253. Quinoa Bowl with Roasted Vegetables:

Cook quinoa according to package instructions. Serve with a side of roasted vegetables (made of cubed sweet potatoes, zucchini, bell peppers, onion, garlic and olive oil).

254. Baked Fish with Asparagus:

Preheat oven to 425°F. Place 2 white fish fillets on a baking sheet. Top with asparagus, olive oil, salt and pepper. Bake for 20 minutes.

255. Grilled Vegetable and Quinoa Salad:

Heat a grill to medium-high heat. Thread bell peppers, zucchini, mushrooms, and onion onto skewers. Grill for 8 minutes, turning occasionally. Serve over cooked quinoa and top with crumbled feta cheese.

256. Baked Eggplant Parmesan:

Cut 2 eggplants into thin slices. Dip in egg whites, then in bread crumbs. Bake at 350°F for 25 minutes. Top with marinara sauce and mozzarella cheese. Bake for an additional 10 minutes.

257. Lentil and Veggie Burgers:

Combine cooked lentils, diced onion, bell peppers, garlic and spices in a bowl. Form into patties and grill. Serve on whole grain buns with lettuce and tomato.

258. Grilled Salmon with Sautéed Spinach:

Grill 2 salmon fillets. Heat olive oil in a skillet and cook a side of spinach. Serve with a lemon garlic sauce.

259. Baked Tofu with Broccoli:

Preheat oven to 400°F. Cut 1 package of extra firm tofu into cubes. Place on a baking sheet. Top with diced broccoli, olive oil, salt and pepper. Bake for 25 minutes.

260. Zucchini Noodles with Avocado Pesto:

Spiralize 2 zucchinis. Toss with avocado pesto (made of avocado, garlic, basil, pine nuts, olive oil, and lemon juice). Top with diced tomatoes and feta cheese.

261. Mediterranean Quinoa Bowl:

Cook quinoa according to package instructions, top with olive oil, diced tomatoes, feta cheese, black olives and parsley.

262. Eggplant and Quinoa Casserole:

Preheat oven to 375°F. Combine cooked quinoa, diced eggplant, diced tomatoes, garlic, and spices in a bowl. Place in a baking dish and top with crumbled feta cheese. Bake for 25 minutes.

263. Baked Cod with Roasted Asparagus:

Preheat oven to 425°F. Place 2 cod fillets on a baking sheet. Top with asparagus, olive oil, salt and pepper. Bake for 20 minutes.

264. Grilled Vegetable Skewers:

Heat a grill to medium-high heat. Thread bell peppers, zucchini, mushrooms, and onion onto skewers. Grill for 8 minutes, turning occasionally.

265. Baked Tilapia with Roasted Tomatoes:

Preheat oven to 450°F. Place 2 tilapia fillets on a baking sheet. Top with diced tomatoes, olive oil, salt and pepper. Bake for 20 minutes.

266. Baked Salmon with Roasted Potatoes:

Preheat oven to 425°F. Place 2 salmon fillets on a baking sheet. Top with cubed potatoes, olive oil, salt and pepper. Bake for 20 minutes.

267. Quinoa and Veggie Stir Fry:

Heat olive oil in a skillet, add diced onion, bell peppers, mushrooms, and garlic. Cook for 5 minutes. Add in cooked quinoa, diced carrots, chopped broccoli and a dash of soy sauce. Cook for another 5 minutes.

268. Turkey Chili:

Cook 1 pound of ground turkey in a large pot. Add diced onion, bell peppers, garlic, chili powder, cumin, oregano, and tomato sauce. Simmer for 20 minutes.

269. Grilled Chicken Salad:

Grill 2 chicken breasts. Cut into cubes and place on a bed of spinach and Romaine lettuce. Top with sliced avocado, diced tomatoes and light vinaigrette.

270. Baked Eggplant with Lentils:

Preheat oven to 375°F. Cut 2 eggplants into cubes. Place on a baking sheet. Top with cooked lentils, olive oil, salt and pepper. Bake for 25 minutes.

271. Lentil Soup:

Heat olive oil in a large pot. Add diced onion, bell peppers, garlic, and spices. Cook for 5 minutes. Add lentils, vegetable broth, and diced tomatoes. Simmer for 30 minutes.

272. Grilled Portobello Mushrooms:

Heat a grill to medium-high heat. Grill 4 portobello mushrooms for 8 minutes, flipping once. Serve with a side of roasted vegetables.

273. Vegetable Curry:

Heat olive oil in a large pot. Add diced onion, bell peppers, garlic, and spices. Cook for 5 minutes. Add diced tomatoes, vegetable broth, and cooked quinoa. Simmer for 20 minutes.

274. Baked Tilapia with Broccoli:

Preheat oven to 450°F. Place 2 tilapia fillets on a baking sheet. Top with diced broccoli, olive oil, salt and pepper. Bake for 20 minutes.

275. Quinoa Bowl with Roasted Vegetables:

Cook quinoa according to package instructions. Serve with a side of roasted vegetables (made of cubed sweet potatoes, zucchini, bell peppers, onion, garlic and olive oil).

276. Baked Salmon with Spinach:

Preheat oven to 425°F. Place 2 salmon fillets on a baking sheet. Top with a side of spinach, olive oil, salt and pepper. Bake for 20 minutes.

277. Baked Tofu with Roasted Vegetables:

Preheat oven to 400°F. Cut 1 package of extra firm tofu into cubes. Place on a baking sheet. Top with roasted vegetables (made of cubed sweet potatoes, zucchini, bell peppers, onion, garlic and olive oil). Bake for 25 minutes.

278. Baked Eggplant with Quinoa:

Preheat oven to 375°F. Cut 2 eggplants into cubes. Place on a baking sheet. Top with cooked quinoa, olive oil, salt and pepper. Bake for 25 minutes.

279. Grilled Shrimp with Roasted Tomatoes:

Heat a grill to medium-high heat. Grill 4 shrimp for 4 minutes, flipping once. Serve with a side of roasted tomatoes (made of diced tomatoes, olive oil, salt and pepper).

280. Lentil and Veggie Burgers:

Combine cooked lentils, diced onion, bell peppers, garlic and spices in a bowl. Form into patties and grill. Serve on whole grain buns with lettuce and tomato.

281. Baked Tofu with Broccoli:

Preheat oven to 400°F. Cut 1 package of extra firm tofu into cubes. Place on a baking sheet. Top with diced broccoli, olive oil, salt and pepper. Bake for 25 minutes.

282. Mediterranean Quinoa Bowl:

Cook quinoa according to package instructions, top with olive oil, diced tomatoes, feta cheese, black olives and parsley.

283. Eggplant and Quinoa Casserole:

Preheat oven to 375°F. Combine cooked quinoa, diced eggplant, diced tomatoes, garlic, and spices in a bowl. Place in a baking dish and top with crumbled feta cheese. Bake for 25 minutes.

284. Grilled Salmon with Sautéed Spinach:

Grill 2 salmon fillets. Heat olive oil in a skillet and cook a side of spinach. Serve with a lemon garlic sauce.

285. Baked Cod with Roasted Asparagus:

Preheat oven to 425°F. Place 2 cod fillets on a baking sheet. Top with asparagus, olive oil, salt and pepper. Bake for 20 minutes.

286. Baked Eggplant Parmesan:

Cut 2 eggplants into thin slices. Dip in egg whites, then in bread crumbs. Bake at 350°F for 25 minutes. Top with marinara sauce and mozzarella cheese. Bake for an additional 10 minutes.

287. Grilled Vegetable Skewers:

Heat a grill to medium-high heat. Thread bell peppers, zucchini, mushrooms, and onion onto skewers. Grill for 8 minutes, turning occasionally.

288. Baked Tilapia with Roasted Tomatoes:

Preheat oven to 450°F. Place 2 tilapia fillets on a baking sheet. Top with diced tomatoes, olive oil, salt and pepper. Bake for 20 minutes.

289. Baked Salmon with Roasted Potatoes:

Preheat oven to 425°F. Place 2 salmon fillets on a baking sheet. Top with cubed potatoes, olive oil, salt and pepper. Bake for 20 minutes.

290. Quinoa and Veggie Stir Fry:

Heat olive oil in a skillet; add diced onion, bell peppers, mushrooms, and garlic. Cook for 5 minutes. Add in cooked quinoa, diced carrots, chopped broccoli and a dash of soy sauce. Cook for another 5 minutes.

291. Turkey Chili:

Cook 1 pound of ground turkey in a large pot. Add diced onion, bell peppers, garlic, chili powder, cumin, oregano, and tomato sauce. Simmer for 20 minutes.

292. Grilled Chicken Salad: Grill 2 chicken breasts.

Cut into cubes and place on a bed of spinach and Romaine lettuce. Top with sliced avocado, diced tomatoes and a light vinaigrette.

293. Baked Eggplant with Lentils:

Preheat oven to 375°F. Cut 2 eggplants into cubes. Place on a baking sheet. Top with cooked lentils, olive oil, salt and pepper. Bake for 25 minutes.

294. Lentil Soup:

Heat olive oil in a large pot. Add diced onion, bell peppers, garlic, and spices. Cook for 5 minutes. Add lentils, vegetable broth, and diced tomatoes. Simmer for 30 minutes.

295. Grilled Portobello Mushrooms:

Heat a grill to medium-high heat. Grill 4 portobello mushrooms for 8 minutes, flipping once. Serve with a side of roasted vegetables.

296. Vegetable Curry:

Heat olive oil in a large pot. Add diced onion, bell peppers, garlic, and spices. Cook for 5 minutes. Add diced tomatoes, vegetable broth, and cooked quinoa. Simmer for 20 minutes.

297. Zucchini Noodles with Avocado Pesto:

Spiralize 2 zucchinis. Toss with avocado pesto (made of avocado, garlic, basil, pine nuts, olive oil, and lemon juice). Top with diced tomatoes and feta cheese.

298. Cauliflower Rice Bowl:

Heat olive oil in a skillet. Add diced onion, bell peppers, garlic, and spices. Cook for 5 minutes. Add riced cauliflower and cook for an additional 5 minutes. Serve with diced tomatoes, black beans, and a light vinaigrette.

299. Baked Sweet Potato Fries:

Preheat oven to 400°F. Cut 2 sweet potatoes into wedges. Toss with olive oil, salt and pepper. Bake for 25 minutes, flipping once.

300. Eggplant and Lentil Curry:

Heat olive oil in a large pot. Add diced eggplant, onion, bell peppers, garlic, and spices. Cook for 5 minutes. Add lentils, diced tomatoes, and vegetable broth. Simmer for 20 minutes.

DESERT

301. Quinoa Salad with Feta and Pomegranate:

Mix together cooked quinoa, feta cheese, pomegranate seeds, fresh parsley, fresh mint, olive oil, lemon juice, and sea salt.

302. Avocado and Mango Salad:

Combine diced avocados, diced mango, red onion, chopped cilantro, lime juice, and a pinch of salt.

303. Grilled Eggplant and Zucchini Skewers:

Cut up eggplant and zucchini into cubes and skewer them onto metal or wooden skewers. Grill for about 10 minutes, or until vegetables are tender. Serve with a side of tzatziki sauce.

304. Stuffed Peppers with Quinoa:

Core bell peppers and fill them with cooked quinoa, diced tomatoes, garlic, onion, and feta cheese. Bake in the oven at 350 degrees for 25 minutes.

305. Grilled Vegetable Platter:

Slice up a variety of vegetables such as eggplant, zucchini, bell peppers, and mushrooms. Grill the vegetables until they are tender and lightly charred. Sprinkle with olive oil, freshly squeezed lemon juice, and sea salt.

306. Chickpea and Spinach Curry:

Saute onions, garlic, and ginger in oil. Add canned chickpeas, diced tomatoes, spinach, and curry powder. Simmer for 15 minutes. Serve with cooked basmati rice.

307. Sweet Potato Fries:

Cut sweet potatoes into 1/4-inch slices. Toss with olive oil and spices. Spread on a baking sheet and bake at 400 degrees for 30 minutes.

308. Mediterranean Baked Fish:

Place a filet of white fish in an oven-safe dish. Top with chopped tomatoes, olives, garlic, oregano, and lemon slices. Drizzle with olive oil and bake at 375 degrees for 20 minutes.

309. Eggplant Parmesan:

Slice an eggplant into 1/4-inch slices. Brush with olive oil and bake at 400 degrees for 15 minutes. Top with marinara sauce and shredded mozzarella cheese. Bake for an additional 10 minutes.

310. Quinoa Pilaf:

Saute onions, garlic, and mushrooms in oil. Add cooked quinoa and vegetable broth. Simmer for 15 minutes. Stir in chopped parsley and season with sea salt.

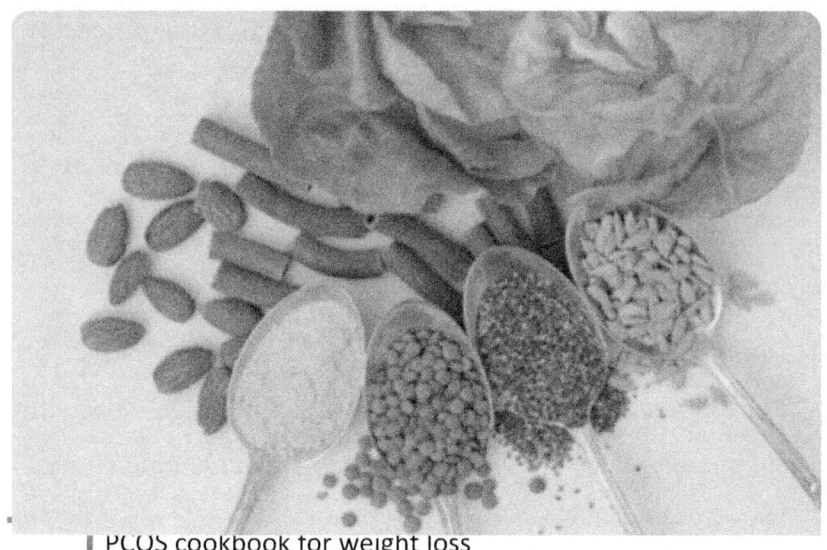

SNACKS

311. Baked Apples with Cinnamon: Core and slice an apple, sprinkle with cinnamon and bake until soft.

312. Avocado Toast with Poached Egg: Toast a piece of whole-grain bread, spread with mashed avocado and top with a poached egg.

313. Kale Chips: Preheat oven to 350°F, coat kale leaves in olive oil and sprinkle with salt. Bake for 10-15 minutes.

314. Baked Sweet Potato Fries: Preheat oven to 425°F. Cut sweet potatoes into wedges. Coat with olive oil and bake for 20 minutes, flipping halfway through.

315. Cucumber Slices with Hummus: Slice cucumber and serve with hummus.

316. Baked Zucchini Coins with Parmesan:

Preheat oven to 400°F. Cut zucchini into slices and coat with olive oil and Parmesan cheese. Bake for 20 minutes.

317. Roasted Chickpeas:

Preheat oven to 400°F. Rinse and drain chickpeas. Toss with olive oil and any desired seasonings. Roast for 20-25 minutes.

318. Greek Yogurt with Berries:

Top a cup of Greek yogurt with fresh or frozen berries.

319. Apple Slices with Almond Butter:

Slice an apple and spread almond butter on top.

320. Celery with Peanut Butter:

Spread peanut butter on slices of celery.

321. Roasted Eggplant Rounds:

Preheat oven to 400°F. Slice eggplant into rounds and coat with olive oil. Bake for 15-20 minutes.

322. Popcorn with Coconut Oil:

Pop popcorn kernels in a pot with coconut oil and sprinkle with desired seasonings.

323. Baked Tofu Fries:

Preheat oven to 425°F. Cut firm tofu into cubes and coat with olive oil and desired seasonings. Bake for 30 minutes, flipping halfway through.

324. Baked Potato Wedges:

Preheat oven to 375°F. Cut potatoes into wedges and coat with olive oil, salt and pepper. Bake for 25 minutes.

325. Baked Kale Chips:

Preheat oven to 350°F. Tear kale leaves into bite-sized pieces and coat with olive oil, salt and pepper. Bake for 10-15 minutes.

326. Avocado Egg Salad:

Mash an avocado and combine with one hard-boiled egg, diced tomatoes, and diced cucumbers.

327. Baked Plantain Chips:

Preheat oven to 350°F. Slice plantains into thin slices and coat with olive oil. Bake for 10-15 minutes.

328. Roasted Cauliflower:

Preheat oven to 400°F. Cut cauliflower into florets and coat with olive oil, salt, and pepper. Roast for 20-25 minutes.

329. Greek Yogurt with Granola:

Top a cup of Greek yogurt with a tablespoon of granola.

330. Zucchini Noodles with Pesto:

Spiralize zucchini and top with store-bought pesto.

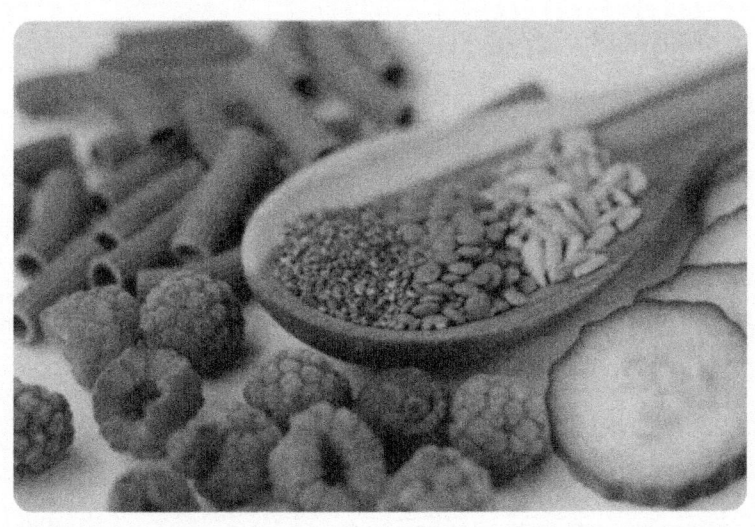

CHAPTER FIVE

Meal Preparation Tips and Strategies

1. Plan ahead: Decide what meals you want to prepare for the week and shop accordingly. Make sure to have plenty of healthy ingredients on hand.

2. Choose healthy ingredients: Focus on lean proteins, complex carbohydrates, and plenty of fresh fruits and vegetables.

3. Utilize your kitchen appliance: Slow cookers, pressure cookers and air fryers are great tools to meal prep with.

4. Make large batches: Make large batches of meals and store them in the refrigerator or freezer for easy access later.

5. Prep ahead: Chop vegetables and measure out ingredients to save time on busy days.

6. Pack meals the night before: Pack meals for the next day the night before so you don't have to worry about it in the morning.

7. Use containers: Use BPA-free containers to store your meal prepped meals.

8. Spice it up: Get creative and use different herbs and spices to make your meal prepped meals more flavorful.

9. Have a variety: Incorporate different types of meals and flavors to keep your meal prepping interesting and enjoyable.

10. Enjoy the process: Meal prepping can be a fun and healthy activity if you allow it to be. Take the time to enjoy the process and experiment with different recipes.

CHAPTER SIX

PCOS friendly exercises for weight loss

1. Walking: Taking a brisk walk for 30 minutes a day is an excellent way to lose weight. Not only does it help you burn calories, but it also helps to reduce stress and balance hormones.

2. Yoga: Yoga is one of the most effective ways to reduce PCOS symptoms, including weight gain. It helps to reduce inflammation, improve digestion, and boost circulation.

3. Cycling: Cycling is a great low-impact exercise that can help with weight loss. It increases heart rate and helps to burn calories while also strengthening muscles.

4. HIIT: High-intensity interval training is an effective way to get your heart rate up and burn calories. Choose

exercises like sprints, burpees, and jumping jacks to get the most out of your workout.

5. Resistance Training: Adding resistance training to your routine can help you build muscle and burn fat. Choose exercises like squats, lunges, and push-ups for a full-body workout.

6. Pilates: Pilates is a great low-impact exercise that helps to build core strength and improve flexibility. It can help to reduce stress and improve overall health.

CONCLUSION

This PCOS Cookbook for Weight Loss has offered a wide range of tasty and healthy recipes that are designed to help those with PCOS lose weight. We hope that you have found useful tips, recipes, and advice to help you reach your weight loss goals. Eating healthy and exercising regularly are essential components of any successful weight loss program. With the right tools and guidance, you can achieve your weight loss goals one step at a time. We wish you the best of luck on your journey to a healthier you!

Printed in Great Britain
by Amazon